THE COMPLETE
GUIDE TO
ORTHODONTIC
ADVERTISING

Find Patients That Pay, Stay and Refer!

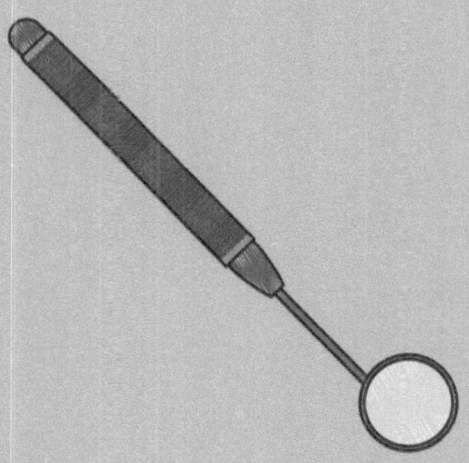

BY ADAM ROSELAND

THE
COMPLETE GUIDE TO
ORTHODONTIC
ADVERTISING

Find Patients That Pay, Stay and Refer!

Adam Roseland

Table of Contents

INTRODUCTION

Running a local orthodontic practice is challenging, even if you've been in business 5-10 years. So many established practices have a few loyal patients but struggle getting new leads on a *consistent* monthly basis. I've worked in digital marketing for more than 15 years and helped over one hundred local businesses dominate online advertising. So many times, I hear clients say they really thought their practice would have grown more in the time they were open.

You likely already know that advertising online will help but there is so much information online saturating the market with various ways to start and grow an orthodontic practice. Even the sites with a special focus on digital marketing "best practices" can all be really overwhelming. While there is likely some value floating around the world wide web, it can be extremely difficult to know which strategies and techniques are the best fit for you.

In this book we are going to cover nine different factors that impact your ability to successfully scale your already steady practice in the coming years. I will cover the problems with traditional marketing, the strategies we use to help our clients get patients who pay, refer and stay for years to come.

CHAPTER 1

THE PROBLEM ORTHODONTISTS FACE WITH TRADITIONAL MARKETING

If I had a dollar for every time one of my clients said they were struggling with getting consistent leads using the marketing strategies they learned in college, I would be able to shut my agency down and retire to a tropical island in the Caribbean. For my clients, money isn't materializing at the mere mention of their antiquated marketing tactics. So, I'll continue to help them modernize and improve their current efforts.

While the chapter title suggests there is only one problem with using traditional marketing in the orthodontic industry, the truth is that there really are many. But for the purposes of this book we are going to focus on three that I think are universal. Of course, identifying the problems is only the first step in many to turning your marketing around and (gasp!) actually making it profitable.

Problem #1: Traditional Marketing Borders on Predatory

There is a reason that the FTC regulates telemarketing and other sales activities. Old-school outbound sales reps created a bad reputation for marketers by aggressively pressuring their leads. Don't get me wrong, it's actually false to say people "don't like to be sold to." Surprisingly, the truth is the opposite. People LOVE to be sold to; they just like to feel like they have control over how it's done.

To really build an incredible marketing strategy, you have to be able to connect with your patients (past, current and future) in a way that builds a trusting relationship. They want to know they aren't just some number on the wall. They need to believe that you have their best interest at heart in any interaction, sales or otherwise. Failing to do so in such a transparency-driven society is almost a death sentence for any business. It just may be a slow and painful one.

When you're simply buying cold emails and making sales calls or emails in bulk for example, there is often no real vetting of the leads which means that so many of your resources are being wasted. Not only that, but you are likely burning bridges that may have otherwise provided an ROI had you used a more progressive approach.

With the technology available today, there isn't a good reason to *avoid* putting effort into being intentional and properly nurturing your potential audience and existing pipeline. YOU know that people in your community need your services. It's not like your practice is new! The trouble is finding a way to stay top of mind so that they don't forget you when they are ready to buy, which actually leads into the next problem we are covering.

Problem #2: Traditional Marketing Doesn't Build Authority the Right Way

I'm sure you've heard the phrase "lead with value" so many times that it likely inspires a deep eye roll. While I try really hard not to ever come across as cliché, I have to admit that it's spot on. The issue is more with identifying what kind of value makes the most sense for the goals you have set for your practice.

Many interpret "providing value" to mean giving something away. But value can come in the form of education, entertainment, network and even tangibles. Yes, people want to be sold to. No, they don't want to be spammed with the exact same pitch over and over when your timing is not right for their needs.

Authority building happens when you put effort into giving them a reason to follow and interact with you *even when they don't need your services*. Of course, we will dive into this in much more detail in the coming chapters but it's important to understand that billboards, radio spots, mailers, cold calls and cold emails just aren't going to set you apart from the competition. The good news is as an established and seasoned orthodontist, you likely have a hotbed of potential business that simply needs to be reactivated and nurtured. You benefit from not having to start from scratch!

Problem #3: It's Not Measurable or Even Consistent

Speaking of billboards, radio and mailers, can I just say let's not? I understand that back in the day, options were pretty limited. But that is not the case anymore. You can be louder, bigger and more visible in a completely different and more intentional way.

The third issue I see with clients using traditional methods is that they just can't track their effectiveness accurately. Very rarely does anyone say they chose their orthodontist because they saw him on a billboard on I-44 or heard her awesome radio ad.

That billboard and radio aren't going to send you a monthly report telling you exactly how many people saw your ad or for how long they listened to your commercial. There is no way to even guarantee that you can get in front of the same people every day. It's subject to the elements and far more distraction than one would have scrolling on social media.

Sure, you can send mailers out to thousands of homes, but you have no way of knowing the percentage of people who that literature was relevant for. After all these years it still amazes me that seasoned business owners are willing to pour enormous amounts of money into a method without knowing the projected return on their investment.

So, Where Do We Go from Here?

That said, I'm not knocking the orthodontists here; the truth is you don't know what you don't know. You spent a lot of money and many years in school to learn the techniques that helped you get to where you are right now. And while you probably aren't 100% happy with where you are (hence reading this book), you can't deny the fact that you have had a level of success to be proud of! Getting off the ground is *sooo* hard and you have stood the test of time, even if it was by a thread.

But the goal is that by the end of this book, you *will* know and be in a better position to grow your practice consistently and sustainably. You will be able to throw out all the dated and ineffective methods, save probably thousands of dollars on "guess" marketing and be able to position yourself as the go-to orthodontist in your community.

In the coming chapters we are going to really dive into creating foundational pieces of your overall marketing plan by giving you a cliff notes guide to help save you the years it took me to learn it all. I know there are so many agencies out there who are overpromising and under delivering on their promises. I'm not one of them. This book isn't theory or concepts I read about once and decided to teach. The things I'm teaching you are born of real-life results that I get every single day from working exclusively with orthodontists.

We do the hard work; we help our clients establish a brand and analyze their audience to ensure that dollars aren't being sunk into guesses. We build their entire marketing strategy from top to bottom and help them get results fast. And since we can't be everywhere and work with everyone at the same time, I wanted to make sure we had the hard lessons documented to allow more orthodontists to experience success and less overall stress.

As we move into the next chapter, I want you to remember that this is not me being critical but an actual effort to help you finally hit the numbers you need and want to hit. So much of it is going to resonate and make sense that you will wonder why you waited to change things up.

Now let's move on to discussing turning a practice into a brand.

CHAPTER 2
TURNING YOUR PRACTICE INTO A BRAND

Most business owners know that having a strong brand is important, but what exactly does it do for an orthodontic practice? When a prospect searches in Google for an orthodontist, there are at times, thousands of local orthodontist listings that come up. SO, you have to ask yourself, what is it about your orthodontic practice website that makes prospects choose you? Personal branding is a powerful way to make you stand out from your competitors. It helps drive more traffic to your website, develop brand recognition and build a stronger patient base to increase your profits.

Why Branding Is Important in Marketing

If you think branding is about having a professional website with a logo and brand colors, you are right, but that's only a small part of it. While there are many orthodontists with the same skill set as you, you are the only orthodontist that is you. A strong brand can go a long way toward establishing your unique place in the local market.

Benefits of Personal Branding for Orthodontists

Imagine for a moment being the orthodontist of choice in your community. You choose who you want to work with, what you want to charge, and where you want to offer your services. Instead of chasing customers, you are attracting patients who resonate with who you are and the way you do business. A powerful brand creates a reputation that precedes you and positions you on top giving you the power to choose.

So how do you begin to go about creating a personal brand that's memorable? *A brand should help a patient determine everything that they need to know about your services at a glance:*

- Who are you?
- What do you do?
- What results should they expect from working with you?
- Why are you different from other orthodontists in your area?

Let's walk through it step by step.

Differentiate yourself. Take a look at the different strengths that your practice has and that your staff can bring to the table. Is there a unique offering that your office performs? Do you offer sedation orthodontics? Do you specialize in pediatric orthodontics? Do you offer holistic services? Perhaps you serve the Latino community? Does a staff member know sign language? Focus on what you do best as well as differently, and you'll attract a strong following.

Personalization. Place bios for the orthodontists and staff on your website. People want to know what's unique about you. What made you get into orthodontics? Are you a Cubs fan? Do you fish in your spare time? Do you regularly compete in marathons? Are you a cancer survivor? The more you share about your personal life, the deeper the connection your customers have with you. When customers feel they have something in common with you or admire what you do, it creates a bond.

Photos. Hire a professional to take photos of your staff and facility, it's worth the investment. Customers want to see what your office looks like. They want to see the orthodontist's staff. Going to the orthodontist can be a scary thing for many customers. Building relationships and trust with photos goes a long way to building comfort for anyone trying a new orthodontist.

Causes. Is your practice involved in any philanthropic efforts? When customers see that you are supporting a cause they are passionate about it makes them feel good about doing business with you. Instead of just being a source for orthodontic services, your business is someone making a difference in the community.

Appearances. Having a brand color scheme uniquely positions your orthodontic firm. For instance, if you are holistic, you may have decor with natural elements and colors. Play relaxing music in the background. Your scrubs can carry across that same theme. Or if you perform children's orthodontics, your office could be decorated in rainbow colors with tie-dye scrubs communicating that same fun theme.

Brand Promise. Your brand should say a lot about your level of skill and the care that you provide for your patients. It's about under-promising and over-delivering. Share that you are kind, gentle, and always put the patient first. Assure them that you use state of the art technologies. Promise to listen to their needs and tailor services. Place your promise on your website. You can also post it on a plaque in your office.

Tagline. Boost your branding with an original tagline to encourage prospective patients. A few examples are: Improving the world, one smile at a time; Family orthodontics with a woman's touch; and Helping keep Portland kids smiling! Notice how each tagline shares some personality and focus on why they are different. Use this on your website and social media pages.

Amenities. Let patients know the extras they can enjoy while being a patient of yours. Do you offer specials for new patients? Do you offer convenient evening hours? Do you have financing options for patients who don't have orthodontic insurance? Sometimes the littlest things make doing business with you the convenient choice.

Consistent Branding is Key

Once you've established a practice brand, use it with every touchpoint the customer has with you. This includes social media, the website, direct mail, how you answer the phone, your decor, your uniforms and more.

Defining your brand as an orthodontic professional can help you find patients and build your reputation. Take the time to invest in creating a brand for your practice and watch your orthodontic career grow.

CHAPTER 3

PROVEN WAYS TO UNDERSTAND *AND* DISCOVER YOUR IDEAL PATIENT

You can be the best orthodontist in the world. You use state of the art equipment, you have an excellent chairside manner, your reputation is impeccable. You have a desirable location with a staff that is second to none. But unless you regularly market your orthodontic practice, your appointment books will be empty.

So, what's the key to attracting people in need of your services so you can focus on providing quality care to your patients?

While it's tempting to think that everyone needs your product or service, in reality, working off this assumption will inevitably lead you down what I call the "make no money" path.

In your attempt to serve everyone, you will end up doing a serious disservice to the people who need you most. The services you deliver won't reach your prospects, and you'll continually find you're attracting the wrong clientele.

Many practices fail at attracting their target audience and turn to the general population out of desperation, thinking they'll have better luck with bigger numbers. But this is any easy way to get lost in the crowd.

Customer profiling can be an invaluable way to target your ideal customers. It helps you pinpoint exactly how to sell and promote the right services to attract your ideal customer. Who are the best patients to do business with and what kinds of things do these people find important? Those are your ideal customers.

Are you an endodontist, orthodontist, pediatric orthodontist, oral surgeon, periodontist, prosthodontist, or cosmetic orthodontist? What are the top three types of orthodontic procedures that you like to perform? It's important to let your customers know what areas of orthodontics you specialize in.

I want to guide you through identifying your ideal customer so that you can enjoy a successful practice.

1. What geographic area do you serve? Name the cities within 10-20 miles of your practice.

2. What is the county your business resides in? Let customers know the major city that your office is near. This is one of the primary ways that people will search for you online to find an orthodontist that is located close to them.

The next step is to create an avatar for your ideal customer. An avatar is a profile of an actual person that represents your ideal client. When you write your marketing communications to a specific individual, it adds warmth and connection to your messaging. Personal communications that feel like they are directly from you to one specific person will outperform a general message every time.

Think about the key demographics of the patients you are trying to help. Identify the age, income, race, gender of your office's target market so that you can focus on marketing to this group. What specific pains and challenges is this person facing? What do they worry about? You should have several profiles which detail different kinds of ideal customers who have certain interests, needs and tendencies, etc. More than one type of person will be purchasing your services, so before you move forward with marketing, you need to hammer out your target profiles.

While you are working on your ideal customer avatar, take a close look at your existing ideal customers. Who are they? How did they find you?

What services of yours do they use? Understanding exactly who you serve helps you understand and shape who you want to serve in the future.

Check your social media responses. What do clients say about you? What about your services stands out in their mind? Why did they choose you? How did they hear about you? Leverage what you learn to help you reach future customers.

Look at all your past marketing efforts and the results. What was a flop? What got a great response? See what clues you can gather from what worked before. The problem we see with many clients is that can't answer these questions definitively because they didn't track their efforts effectively, an essential part of successful advertising.

Spy on your competitors to see what you can learn. Find out on what page they rank in Google. Review their website and social media channels to see who they are serving, the messages they use, and what is working for them. Just do so with caution, looks can sometimes be deceiving.

Market your orthodontic services using what you've learned. Your research should have revealed where your target audience hangs out online. You should have learned more about what is important for them in choosing an orthodontist. Use this information to streamline your marketing efforts. By developing and maintaining long-term satisfying relationships with your patients, you'll create a thriving orthodontic practice.

If you are you ready to grow your practice and help more patients, defining who your ideal customers are will help you target your marketing moving forward. Each profile of an ideal patient will help you figure out what will ultimately make that customer choose your company over the competition.

CHAPTER 4

ORTHODONTIC MARKETING STARTER KIT

A s an orthodontist, marketing is a **continuous** need for your business. It's important to constantly be working on ways to stay ahead of your competition and generate new leads. It used to be that the yellow pages brought you business. But these days if you aren't marketing online, you are falling behind.

When making decisions about how to invest your time and online marketing dollars, there are a few important distinctions to consider. Such as *where are you now* in your business? Is your practice stagnant or shrinking? Are you growing and want to continue momentum? Whatever your situation, if you can use more patients you're in luck. I am going to share what I consider an "orthodontist marketing starter kit" or basic things you need to advertise your practice successfully using local SEO, Google Ads, Facebook Ads, and retargeting and break them down further in the coming chapters.

Local SEO

Your orthodontic website plays an important role in attracting new patients. It also determines how easy your website is to find in the search engines. Today there are a lot of orthodontists in your area vying for the same patients. When a patient is looking for an orthodontist in their area, they will do a Google search from their phone or laptop typing "orthodontist near me" or something similar. Whether you come up on the first page of Google in that search is important. That's where local SEO comes in.

Imagine doing research that tells you the top phrases that new patients in your area are using online to search for new orthodontists, then knowing how to plug those keywords into your website in a way that converts more leads.

Once you know those keywords you can write blog articles around them. You can optimize your website for them. Writing blog articles helps you rank higher on Google, Yahoo, & Bing. It positions you as the top orthodontist in your area. Your SEO optimized articles just keep attracting more and more traffic over time.

For example, if a new patient is searching for information about Invisible Aligners and they type in the phrase "cost of invisible aligners," if you have written a blog post on the cost of invisible aligners, then Google will see the match, recognize your original content and boost the ranking of your blog.

You can get high quality inbound links from high ranking websites to help boost your authority in the search engines. Google has used inbound links as a primary factor in ranking.

But it's not just about setting it and forgetting it. Local SEO requires constant checking and tweaking. While you may rank on top one day, you can drop to the 2nd or 3rd page of Google results the next. So, it's important to use Google analytics to see what keywords are driving your traffic, which search engines bring you the most visitors, and other key factors.

To rank for any keyword, it requires a lot of perseverance, quality original articles and backlinks. And even then, it takes a while for them to gain the necessary authority.

While you can try to do local SEO on your own, I wouldn't recommend it. SEO rules change frequently. With every Google algorithm update, you have to reevaluate your game. It requires constant training to stay on top of things. Plus, the tools you need to quickly monitor and tweak SEO make the process a whole lot easier than doing it by hand.

One smart use for SEO is lead generation. You can discover topics your patients want to know about and make a free guide they can get by opting in. Then SEO optimize your landing page so that it ranks high in the search engines for that term. When new leads land on this page and sign up for the free report, you can capture their contact information and continue to market to them till they book an appointment. SEO brings a stream of leads to your website, making your website one of the best lead generation tools you have. Another great way to target the interest of a lead visiting your website is to present geo-specific messaging that relates to their residential location. Your website can share specific messaging that is related to their locale.

An orthodontic SEO professional can help you attract and convert more patient leads. They can help you grow your orthodontic practice through customized local search strategies. If you want to dominate your local market and get more patients, local SEO can help you achieve that.

Want to work with me? Book your call at the link below, and if you work with us, mentioning this book will get you $100 towards our services. https://orthoadvertising.com/book-a-call

Google Ads

Have you heard about pay per click marketing? PPC ads like Google Ads are paid online advertisements which appear under or next to relevant searches and other content on the web. Basically, you set up an advertising campaign that you only pay for when a visitor clicks on the ad to visit your website. Google Ads is the single most popular PPC advertising system in the world.

The benefits of Google Ads Campaigns.

1. Let's you reach customers more immediately (faster than SEO).

2. Boosts top-of-mind awareness for your brand.

3. Drives visitors to your website.

4. Measure your performance consistently.

5. Adjust your ads anytime to reach a specific group of people (by interest, geographical area, etc.) or promote a specific service.

6. They're scalable. Once you get an ad that gets high conversions, you can pour more money into your budget and boost your lead conversions.

7. Ability to reach potential customers with Gmail. Google integrated native Gmail ads with Google AdWords.

8. Use of Geotargeting to target your ads to only appear to customers in a certain location(s) that you specify.

9. Turn campaign on and off whenever you want. Turn it on and it's like turning on a faucet and sending new patients to your business. Getting overbooked? Turn the ad off.

But there is a lot more to doing an effective Google Ad campaign then just typing in some words, uploading an image, and setting a campaign budget. You really have to do some research to find the best keywords to optimize lead conversion. You can review your Google Analytics to see:

- Who clicked on your ad
- How many leads were generated
- How much traffic the ad sent to your website
- Which keyword generated the most traffic and leads
- What the cost per lead was

Here are a few Google ad basics to keep in mind. Make the landing pages that visitors are sent to super relevant to the content of the ad. For instance, if you say "Low cost invisible aligners" on the ad and send traffic to your general orthodontic services page, that is not relevant.

Optimize for Negative Keywords. Look for any words that are getting a lot of clicks, but not many conversions. You can remove anything that's getting high impressions and low clicks. By narrowing your match type for the ad, you'll get more relevant impressions, but decreased volume. That means you pay less but get more relevant leads.

Some other Ad optimization techniques include using the correct keyword match types, adjusting bids for geotargeting, breaking out mobile-optimized campaigns and more.

The task of managing an effective Google Ads campaign can be quite challenging. Orthodontic practices have marketing budget challenges and many orthodontists lack the proper knowledge of Google Ads. Most orthodontists don't have the time to track, monitor and adjust a Google Ads campaign. They don't know the proper keywords to use. Plus, they don't have copywriting or graphic design expertise to create an effective ad. In the Google Ads world, a mistake can cost you big time. A poorly designed campaign can cost you a ton in clicks but send poor quality traffic that's not a match.

A well optimized Google Ads campaign can bring you more quality patients and maximum revenue for your practice. Working with an orthodontic marketing firm can ensure Google Ads expertise, orthodontic industry knowledge, and exceptional ad campaign performance. Plus, your practice will achieve better results for Google Ads campaigns while saving a lot of money.

Want to work with me? Book your call at the link below, and if you work with us, mentioning this book will get you $100 towards our services. https://orthoadvertising.com/book-a-call

Facebook Ads

Like Google Ads, Facebook Ads are a pay per click advertising option for your orthodontic practice. Facebook ads can target users based on their location, demographic, and profile information.

Facebook is the perfect platform to advertise your orthodontic services. Facebook is continually growing in usage. Currently with over 2.6 billion monthly active Facebook users, Facebook is the largest and most powerful social media advertising platform in the world. It's really important before starting a pay per click campaign to evaluate who your ideal customers are and what social platforms they are on.

Here's some best practices for Facebook Ads:
- Target your ads to your orthodontic practice's target audience.
- Make your ad copy personal to speak to your ideal client.
- Test your calls to action with A/B testing.
- Try several ad types to see what pulls best.
- Feature your orthodontic practice staff in your ads.
- Design holiday and seasonal ad campaigns.
- Create new patient ads to people who have recently moved.
- Offer a free gift with a visit.

Why Facebook Ads Perform Poorly

On average, 80% of potential conversions from Facebook are lost to poor ad strategy. To succeed with Facebook Ads, you need to understand how to drive user engagement and effectively use audience targeting to get the most out of your advertising budget.

Facebook allows you to target audiences using categories like age, gender or interests to yield best results. In addition,, you can build custom audiences to really get the most out of your campaigns. You can even upload your customer list to help target the right future customers. That makes it easy to identify and attract new traffic with high conversion potential.

Testing and tweaking your ads are the second half of the battle. You need several versions of ads to test and see what works best. Having a relevant landing page is equally important. If you have a high converting ad and send them to a low converting landing page, you've lost the lead. So, it's really important to make sure the ad and the landing page are highly targeted. Then you need to check and adjust ads regularly to ensure best ad performance. Knowing Facebook statistics and trends can help you modify your Facebook Ad strategy so that you can increase engagement, reach your audience and meet your business goals.

Facebook ads give business owners the power to finely target and reach a specific consumer market, all without breaking the bank on their marketing budget. If you want to get more traffic, acquire more patients and sell more services, consider working with a Facebook Ad professional. They handle everything from research and laser targeting your ideal customer to developing the ad creatives.

Retargeting Ads

Wouldn't it be amazing if when a customer browsed your website and didn't book an appointment that you could still keep in touch and market to them? Retargeting helps you do just that. Have you ever been shopping for shoes on Amazon.com and then gone on Facebook and noticed that all the ads you see are about shoes? That's no coincidence. Retargeting allows you to follow prospective patients around on the web and show ads to them about your orthodontic practice.

Retargeting can lift ad engagement rates up to 400%. 20% of marketers have a budget specifically for retargeting. 25% percent of individuals say they like retargeting ads because they remind them of what they were looking at previously.

This tagging and tracking technique overcomes the problem of someone landing on your website and then never hearing from them again because they haven't left their contact details.

Remarketing is possible with Google Ads and Facebook Ads. The rule of seven says that most people don't buy the first time they come across an offer. You may need to get in front of a prospective patient 7 times before they convert. Remarketing takes advantage of this by continuing to market to them. When you know your market and can reach them with multiple impressions you radically increase your chances of getting a new patient.

Best Practices for Effective Ad Campaigns

When you're pursuing people who have already been to your site, they're perfect targets! Here are a few best practices.

Send remarketing campaigns that are proven and top performing. That gives you the best chance of converting the lead.

Offer special deals to people who leave your site. Think "don't go" or "wait there's more." You can offer them a free cleaning. Try giving a free gift card. Up the ante to make them want to give you a try.

Don't be afraid to spend a little more for remarketing. Once a lead is warm, it's more likely to convert. Chase down these customers.

Common Remarketing Mistakes

Stalking your prospects: Place an impression cap so that your warm leads are not bugged too many times. You don't want to bombard them so many times with ads that they are turned off to your brand.

Just selling: One reason that your prospects left your website might be that they haven't found what they were looking for. So cross sell and upsell.

Many remarketing campaigns are suffering from poor execution and are not producing volume or results like they could with a few best practices applied.

Are you searching for the best marketing companies for orthodontists? If you'd like to generate quality new orthodontic patients for your practice on a consistent basis, finding a professional orthodontic marketing agency can help increase your new patient base and grow your revenue by getting your orthodontic marketing right.

I just happen to know a guy that would be perfect to work with ☺. Book your call at the link below, and if you work with us, mentioning this book will get you $100 towards our services. https://orthoadvertising.com/book-a-call

CHAPTER 5

HOW PATIENTS SEARCH LOCALLY FOR ORTHODONTISTS

L et's dig deeper into how SEO can help your practice. 73% use online search engines to research orthodontic treatments, and the first step 72% of patients take when searching for a new doctor or orthodontist is looking up online reviews. So, if customers can't find you easily online, they'll go to someone they can. Below you'll find the best local search engine optimization ideas for orthodontists that are proven to snag you more new patients.

Organic search results can drive up to 94% of all traffic to websites. That's why a great local SEO strategy is important to drive high-quality leads to your business. Whatever stage your orthodontist practice is in, local search optimization plays a huge part in making it easy for your clients to find you online. Focusing on local patients who live close to your office is a focused, easy way to grow your business. So, if you haven't optimized your business for Google local search, you are failing to take advantage of this significant opportunity. But how do you find these local clients online? The easiest way is local SEO.

Did you know that the first local search engine listing can get over 30% of all search-related traffic, with the top three listings pulling in a combined total of 60% of all traffic? Local SEO is the process of optimizing your website so that it appears in the first positions of Google, Bing and Yahoo for searches that are related to your area / city / county. This means that it is important to make sure that the website shows up in all local searches.

When someone is looking for an orthodontist, they search Google for orthodontist near me/close by, orthodontist Schaumburg, orthodontist northwest suburbs, orthodontist DuPage county or orthodontist Chicago. If customers search for something local, 72% of them will visit the store within five miles of where they are. So, it's important to be found in the search engines by patients who are looking for an office close to them.

Fortunately, local search engine optimization can optimize your website, so your orthodontist practice ranks high in Google, Bing, Yahoo, and other search engines. By increasing your visibility on search engines like Google, it makes it easier to find your website. Additionally, you can use retargeting ads to bring previous website visitors back to your site.

A web developer or search engine marketing firm can optimize your website to boost its visibility in the search engines. After doing keyword research they can format your meta tags. They can optimize your images to load quickly. Plus, they can ensure that your business name, address and phone number are on every page. These key changes inside the coding of your website will make a huge difference in helping local customers find you online.

Update and Optimize Your Google My Business Page.

Having a listing here means that your business is found locally by people in your area. People prefer to frequent an orthodontist that is close to them.

With a Google My Business account, your free business profile lets you easily connect with customers across Google Search and Maps. A complete Google business listing will average 7x more traffic than an empty one. So, it's important to fill out the listing in complete detail to reap the full benefits. That includes adding your

business's categories (either "orthodontist" or "orthodontic practice"), main phone number, business's description, hours of operation, your address and service area, photos, and your review section.

How to Create and List Your Google My Business listing

On your computer, go to Google and search for Google My Business. Click on the link, and then the top-right corner, click Sign in. Sign into your Google Account, or create one. Then, click Next. Enter your business address. You may also be asked to position a marker on the location of your chain's branch on a map.

Choose if you want your business location to appear on Google Maps. Once a new Google My Business listing is created, a Google Maps location is then generated that synchronizes with traditional Google Search for easy access and searchability. Being listed in Google Maps is a great advantage for your business.

Google Maps is utilized by 86% of people to look up a local business. When someone looks for an orthodontist near them, Google Maps will quickly populate with dozens of red markers, showing local orthodontists. This is a great benefit that allows users to instantly see how close you are to where they live, increasing the likelihood that they'll pay you a visit.

Encourage and Record Reviews

Reputation is really important when patients are researching a new orthodontist to try. For new orthodontist customers, one of the biggest hurdles they have to face is that of building enough trust to confidently become a patient. As a practice owner, your job is to help them make that jump as easily as possible. Being highly ranked in the search engines brings some credibility with it. Plus, it gives new customers a chance to check you out first before your competitors.

Positive Google reviews are critical to your success at attracting new patients to your practice. Getting Google Reviews for your practice helps boost your website rankings as well. 97% of consumers are influenced by reviews, with 88% trusting online reviews to make a purchase or contract a service. Plus, the more positive reviews you have, the more clicks it will trigger to your website. In turn, that popularity boosts your website rankings. Ask for customer reviews. After a patient comes in for a visit, send them an email asking for their feedback.

"Hello, we appreciate the trust you place in us for your orthodontic services and we value you as a patient, so we want to know how your appointment went. The greatest compliment you could offer us is a review on our Google Local page. Thanks for sharing your feedback here." *LINK*

Ensure a Mobile friendly website experience

88% of consumer based, local business searches on a mobile device either call or visit the business within 24 hours. If your website doesn't have a responsive design that displays correctly on smart phones, then you are missing out on a lot of traffic. Mobile web design lets your website detect the size of the device that someone is using. Then, your website automatically scales to the size of that device's screen, if you're using responsive design.

Getting a listing in orthodontist directories can also help you be seen. These sites offer ratings and reviews for orthodontist practices near the patient. They can browse the database to find top-rated orthodontists in their local area.

Consider Blogging

Blogging is one of the easiest ways to boost your search engine rankings. Patients are searching for the answers to everything, from how often they need to brush to what kind of toothbrush they should use. Friendly, informative blog posts can help hesitant patients feel more comfortable with your practice. They can also help you establish credibility and show patients that you're the expert in your field. It's a good idea to write 2 to 3 blogs per week. You can also share your blog posts as part of your social media presence, encouraging interaction and engagement with patients.

Write about answers to common orthodontic problems such as gum disease, cavities and tooth sensitivities. Blog about basic orthodontic hygiene like fluoride, cavity protection and mouthwash. Answer questions about non-orthodontic procedures like filling cavities and root canals. Share updates in orthodontic tools and technology that you are using for patients. Explain about teeth whitening. Debunk popular myths about tooth care. If you brainstorm and make a list of topics you'd like to write about, you'll always be ready to go.

Create Backlinks from Authority Websites

Acquiring backlinks for your orthodontic practice website is an important step. Backlinks are references to your website pages from other websites. Getting other websites to link to you improves your site's rankings in search engine results pages. For example, if you are a member of the local Chamber of Commerce and they give you a listing on their website that links to your orthodontic website, that's a backlink.

The best advantage of local SEO is that once you achieve high rankings it can continue to drive free traffic to your website. You don't have to pay for advertising. Just sit back and watch your appointment book fill up.

Once you have identified the geographic regions you want to target, you can make improvements to your existing site to help you rank better in the search engines. Once you have optimized your website, it's important to monitor it to make sure that your site continues to maintain its rankings. When you actively review your website performance you can identify how to adjust your SEO strategy in order to maximize your return.

Are you ready to grow your practice and help more patients? Local SEO has a ton of benefits to your orthodontic practice. With the right website set up and SEO strategy you can boost your bookings and grow your practice.

CHAPTER 6

CREATING YOUR RETIREMENT PLAN
(*AKA GETTING PATIENTS ON DEMAND*)

Retirement planning for orthodontists starts with building a better practice. As orthodontists, we need to challenge ourselves not to only invest our time and energy into our patients but also our practice's profitability. To live the lives we want in retirement, we need to start planning and growing our practice starting today.

Want to know how to grow your orthodontic practice year after year? Building a profitable practice is a three-part process. First, you need to attract clients. Next, you need to give clients an amazing experience to build customer loyalty. Finally, you want to keep them as lifelong clients. (*Pay, stay and refer.*)

To start getting patients on demand, you need a solid marketing plan. Look at what promotions you'll be offering for the year. Then map out content to align with those promotions. That way you aren't scrambling about what to talk about. All your marketing messages and content will be planned in perfect alignment. This includes blog articles, social posts, website updates, email marketing, advertising and contests.

Once you have attracted your ideal patient, you have to deliver exceptional service to keep them. Every touch point you have with your patient makes an impression. It's about how the receptionist treats them when they call with a question or to book an appointment. It's about the first impression they get when they walk in your office and experience the atmosphere and decor. You want to create a comfortable, easy experience for the patient during the orthodontic visit.

Make sure the hygienist is friendly and pain free while cleaning teeth. Stay cutting edge with orthodontic technology so the patient has a great experience with their procedures. Then send them home feeling good about visiting your office.

Let's dive a little deeper into specifics of attracting first time patients. Briefly, let's recap the essential parts of your marketing plan from the previous chapters.

Website

Your website is the modern business card and it reflects who you are in every way. Most patients who are searching for an orthodontist in their area will do a Google search for orthodontists near their home. If your website doesn't come up on the first page of results, they may never see you.

Once prospects do find your website, it's important to make a great first impression. Trying a new orthodontist can be scary, so building trust and credibility with your website is crucial. Your website should look friendly and professional. Include pictures of your office and your staff.

Include your phone number and address on every page. List what procedures you offer in your practice. Share customer reviews. Make it easy for them to book appointments. Share what types of insurance and payments you accept. Mention if you offer flexible payment options. Offer a mailing list sign up. Add links to your social media channels too. Basic website pages include Home, About, Services, FAQ, and Contact.

Branding

Patients are wondering why they should choose you over other orthodontists. Branding is everything when it comes to orthodontic practice marketing. But branding is not just about having a unique logo, tagline or eye-catching graphic design. It's about who you are and how your patients perceive you. Do you specialize in a special procedure? What exceptional results do you create? What do you stand for? What are your values? Once you discover the heart of your brand, make sure your marketing materials are focused on this.

Another part of branding is visual consistency. A brand style guideline should include a comprehensive visual identity to guide content creation, including colors, logos, fonts, photos and illustrations. This ensures that everything from your brochures to social posts have the same look and feel.

SEO

SEO can drive a consistent stream of new patients who are looking for the orthodontic services you provide. Patients turn to search engines first when seeking orthodontic services. You need to be on the first page to get found. SEO can increase your search engine rankings, boost organic search visitors, and increase appointment bookings.

The search engines automatically look for certain keywords in a website to establish relevance to a given search. Search engine optimization gets you in front of potential patients and boosts your overall practice growth.

Online Reviews

Reviews are increasingly more important. It used to be word of mouth that drove patients to try new orthodontists. Today individuals look at online reviews when choosing an orthodontist. The major online review sites are Google Reviews, Facebook Reviews and Yelp.

It's important to provide exceptional service that leads to good reviews. You need to ask clients and tell them how to leave reviews. You also need to perform reputation management by reviewing online reviews. In the case that there is a negative review, you have a chance to respond. It's also possible to hire a review management company to remove a negative review.

Additional Strategies to Use in Your Advertising

Press Releases

If you want more exposure for your orthodontic practice, media exposure is a great way to go. The local media is always looking for stories to share about local businesses. The biggest challenge is finding something newsworthy to share. Does your practice have a new cutting-edge technology? Did your practice celebrate an exciting milestone? Do you have a fun seasonal promotion? Are you doing something to tie into a national holiday? Submit a press release with a picture to your local newspaper. There's nothing like being featured in the local news to get the community talking about you.

Pay Per Click

Doctors who want more leads, more patients and more growth should invest in pay per click advertising. You can run pay per click ads on Google Ads, Bing Ads and Facebook Ads to generate leads.

Geofencing

Geofencing is a mobile service that triggers an action when a smart phone enters a set location. Imagine someone driving by your orthodontic office getting a coupon or text message sent right to their phone.

Retargeting

Remarketing is a form of online advertising that can help you keep your brand in front of bounced traffic after they leave your website. Only a handful of consumers will turn into patients immediately after visiting your website. Retargeting enables ads for your orthodontic practice to follow them around online after they've left your website. For example, imagine someone was browsing for an orthodontist in San Francisco and stumbled across a landing page on your website. He was looking at the teeth whitening services you offer but leaves your site without reaching out to your practice to make an appointment. A retargeting ad is specifically shown to the ones that got away. It's such a smart use of advertising dollars.

Referrals

Gaining new patients through referrals is one of the most effective ways to build your practice, but referrals don't come automatically—you need a system in place. Getting referrals starts with providing a great patient experience. One so amazing they want to tell family, friends and colleagues about your practice. Pick a moment when you know the patient is happy and when you've achieved great results. Sincerely say to the individual that you like having them as a patient and that you would love it if they'd send their friends because you know they'd be great patients, too.

You can also set up a referral system with doctors whose services compliment but don't compete with yours. For example, an orthodontist may want to share referrals with a *pediatric* orthodontist or an oral surgeon. Have a line on the intake form that asks how the patient heard about you. Contact these referring doctors and get a formal referral system in place.

Social Media

Social media can help you reach, engage and increase your patient count to your practice. Choose the social media platforms where you patients visit online. Set yourself apart by sharing smart, useful information for your patients. This builds trust and keeps you at the top of readers' minds when it comes time for them to find a new doctor or make an appointment.

Facebook posting allows you to engage with patients. Create a Facebook cover image that has your phone number on it. List your business location, address and business hours. Optimize your Facebook Business Page for Facebook searches. That way your page is easily found on Facebook when someone searches.

Special Offers

Consider offering a special for new patients. Whether a patient is new to town, needs to try a new orthodontist, or is looking for a more convenient orthodontist, a New Patient Offer is a great introduction to your practice. This could include a free consultation. It could be a free orthodontic exam for new patients. You could offer a low-cost tooth whitening procedure.

Email Marketing

If you are not already doing it, your orthodontic practice needs to embrace email marketing. Email marketing has one of the highest returns on investments (ROI) of all online marketing activities. Email marketing keeps you top of mind with existing patients. It allows you to share valuable information with your patients. You can offer a reward to patients who refer new patients to you. Plus, you can share information on news and updates in the practice.

Video Marketing

If you want to ease new patients' minds, a website video is the perfect way to do it. Imagine sharing a video about what patients can expect when they visit. They can explain to patients about their orthodontic approach, personal and professional background and the nuances of orthodontic practice.

Blogging

If you're an orthodontist thinking about blogging, it is a powerful tool to increase your visibility and help attract new patients. Creating blog posts can help grow your orthodontic practice by positioning you as a thought leader, improving search rankings, and attracting new patients.

Community Involvement

Getting involved in your community can be a great way to give back, as well as raise awareness of your practice and bring patients to your door. You can donate to silent auctions. Get involved in community organizations like Kiwanis, Rotary or Lions Clubs. You'll make your community better while helping your practice grow through networking, all at the same time.

Other community service opportunities are available with Habitat for Humanity, churches, food pantries, soup kitchens, and homeless shelters. There are endless options for community service work, but you should find a project that fulfills you and motivates you to continue your work in the community.

Patient Loyalty Programs

As an orthodontist, your patients are your greatest advocates and the best resource you have to grow your practice. Patient loyalty starts with patient satisfaction which in turn leads to referrals and growth for your practice. Loyalty is not something that can be bought from patients. It's something earned over time, and it starts with the patient experience.

A patient loyalty program is an offering put into place to keep orthodontic patients coming back to your practice and get more patients in the process. You can offer incentives to patients, like a free toothbrush or 15% off their next appointment. Reward clients for booking appointments, giving referrals or purchasing items with a reward card they can redeem at your office for merchandise.

If you want to acquire more patients and become the orthodontic authority in your market, orthodontic marketing helps you fill your practice. Doing the right things in your orthodontic practice today can help you plan for retirement tomorrow.

CHAPTER 7
SURVIVING GOOGLE'S TREACHEROUS ALGORITHM

New patients are the lifeblood of your business but finding them can be hard. That's where Google's algorithm comes in. As an orthodontist, you know that the easier it is for patients to find you in the search engines, the more bookings you will receive. Local search engine optimization is the key to ensuring your orthodontic website gets high rankings. But the fact is that you may rank #1 in Google one day, and #20 the next if Google updates it's algorithm. So what is Google's algorithm and why does it matter to you? See below to find out more.

According to Search Engine Journal, "Google's algorithms are a complex system used to retrieve data from its search index and instantly deliver the best possible results for a query." Basically, that means that Google periodically changes its rules on what criteria it uses to determine how high things rank in their search engine. What this means to you is that you could rank on top one day and slip in rankings the next.

Google's algorithm does the work for you by searching out Web pages that contain the keywords you used to search, then assigning a rank to each page based on several factors, including how many times the keywords appear on the page. When you search for "Chicago orthodontist," Google's algorithm does the work of determining which websites are the best fit for those keywords.

The most important part of Google algorithm's is the PageRank system that determines where each search result appears on Google's search engine return page. PageRank reviews each web page and gives it a score. The higher the page score, the higher the page ranks for a given keyword or phrase. The factors that determine Google PageRank are constantly changing and evolving.

One of the factors that PageRank uses to determine the score of a page is how long a web page has been around. Older pages rank more highly because they have been around for a while.

Another factor influencing PageRank is how many high-ranking sites link to your website. This acts as a score for reputation and popularity to Google PageRank.

Having unique content is also very important. If you post the exact same article on your website, LinkedIn, and an orthodontic association blog, the one on your website will not rank as high. It's better to post unique versions of the website on every place you post it.

Keyword density is another key factor. You don't want to have a keyword density of more than 3%. If you do, it's considered keyword stuffing and seen as manipulative for the purpose of high PageRank. Therefore, checking the keyword density for a given keyword phrase is important so you don't receive penalties.

Social media mentions can boost your PageRank as well. You can post links to blog articles on your profile. When fans comment and your company comments back, that adds a boost. Having lots of tweets about your orthodontic practice can boost your authority in the search engines.

There are a lot of places you can put keywords on your website to help Google determine how well your website matches with the keyword phrase that was searched for. It looks at the page URL, heading, sub headers, page link text, bolded text, underline text and alt tags on images.

When you work with a search engine optimization firm, they will do research to determine which keywords get high traffic with low competition. Finding those keyword phrases is the best strategy for ranking on top.

A Google Algorithm by Any Other Name Doesn't Rank the Same

Every time Google releases a new algorithm; they give it a new name. Below are the names of a few Google Algorithm updates they have released over the years.

- Fred
- Intrusive Interstitials Update
- Mobilegeddon
- RankBrain
- Panda
- Penguin
- Hummingbird
- Pigeon
- Payday
- EMD (Exact Match Domain)
- Page Layout Algorithm

Google is rolling out a new Algorithm update as this is being written. For this update, Google suggests focusing on ensuring you're offering the best content you can. This means original content, that's substantive, with insightful analysis and appropriate title and header tags. Make sure it's free from spelling and grammar errors. It should provide clear value to the readers of your website. Google checks for expertise, authoritativeness and trustworthiness.

DIY SEO

Let's say that you or one of your office staff is going to tackle search engine optimization for your orthodontic practice. Here are some of the things you need to consider.

You need to do keyword research to determine how your best customers are finding you and get a strategy for high search terms that are easier to rank for. Usually this is a long tail term. A short tail term is a brief keyword like Chicago orthodontist. A long tail term is advanced orthodontic care Chicago, IL. There are keyword research tools to help you determine the best phrases to target.

Research your competitors. Find out what phrases they rank for. See what they did to get ranked highly for those phrases. There are spy tools that help you see what paid and organic traffic your competitors are ranking for.

Look for content gaps. See if there are high ranking blog articles your competitor has that you could write and rank for. For example, if your competitor has a 1200-word blog article on best teeth whiteners that ranks on the first page of Google, that represents an opportunity for you to write an original article on the same content and potentially rank high as well.

Review Google Analytics to see how the Local SEO changes you have made are impacting your traffic and conversions.

DIY SEO Mistakes

Search engine optimization is a lot of work. If you try DIY SEO you can mess up what it took someone weeks or months to achieve in terms of high rankings with Google's Algorithm.

You do not have an SEO friendly website.

You have stolen content from another website. Original articles always rank the highest. Never "borrow" an article from another website. Write your own.

You are guilty of keyword stuffing.

In hopes of ranking too high you use your keyword phrase too heavily (more than 3%) and the search engines penalize you.

Avoid the Dreaded Blackhat SEO

There's a dark side to SEO. There are rules to what you can and can't do to rank higher in the search engines. If you are caught doing these things, Google will penalize or even ban you from the search engines. Therefore, knowing what NOT to do is crucially important. Examples include:

- Paying for a link from a high PageRank website to artificially boost your rankings.
- Adding spam comments with your website link on other website blogs to boost your rankings.
- Copying content from another website.
- Using invisible text on a page. For instance, you could put a bunch of white text on the bottom of a white page with keywords solely for the purpose of boosting your rankings.
- Using article spinning to create different versions of the same article. - Article spinning is the process of rewriting an article to create new "original" copies in an attempt to avoid duplicate content issues that can result in a penalty from search engines

- SEO Cloaking - According to Wikipedia "Cloaking is a search engine optimization (SEO) technique in which the content presented to the search engine spider is different from that presented to the user's browser. This is done by delivering content based on the IP addresses or the User-Agent HTTP header of the user requesting the page."

If the traffic of your website has suffered a sudden drop and the ranking has been diminished, it may be because you have received a sanction from Google.

Why You May Want to Call in the Google Algorithm Experts

It's smart for orthodontists to hire an expert who can stay on top of the rapid search engine optimization changes so that their orthodontic practice remains high in Google searches.

Local search engine optimization is a science. Having the tools and knowledge to be effective at SEO requires constant updates and training. It requires consistent review of your rankings and analysis to identify what needs tweaking. What worked in early in the year may be totally different with the new Google algorithm updates that come throughout the year. Always stay on top of algorithm updates.

Effective SEO strategies to keep up with and rank high with Google's algorithm updates requires many different skills and techniques. You have to do on-site optimization, external optimization, meta tags, keywords research, optimizing content, image optimization, mobile SEO, local SEO and voice SEO.

It's important to find someone who has Local SEO experience in your industry. They can grow your orthodontic practice with local targeting, technology, and marketing expertise. They will have experience developing orthodontic-specific strategies that are proven to perform.

They can perform an analysis to show you where your patients are coming from and which neighborhoods produce your highest marketing ROI. Then they can perform a detailed website analysis and search engine ranking report, which uncovers your website strengths and weaknesses.

They can prepare a strategic SEO marketing plan for you. It is a long-term solution to drive pre-qualified traffic to your website, improve conversion rates and boost your online revenue.

They can optimize for voice search. Google Voice Search is a function that allows users to search the Web using Google through spoken voice commands rather than typing.

Voice search is changing the way Google handles search queries and how users search for the information we need. Google Voice Search can be used on both desktop and mobile searches.

Mobile searches are over 50% of all searches, especially for local businesses. This means they aren't talking in their phone using the generic orthodontic terms like Portland orthodontist. They're adding many more qualifying words to their search to get the best results, and to avoid wasting their valuable time.

Plus, an orthodontic SEO agency has data analytics and reporting tools to perform real-time performance management. They can keep a steady watch on your rankings and make key adjustments to keep top rankings.

Factors Determining orthodontic SEO Pricing

With local SEO, you truly get what you pay for, but there can be a lot of factors determining what your SEO services will cost.

Before an orthodontic SEO firm works with you, they will want to perform an analysis to see how well SEO-optimized your website currently is. They will:

1. Review how competitive it is for orthodontists in your geographic area.
2. Determine how well you are ranking in Google now.
3. See how well your website is currently SEO optimized.
4. Check how much original content is on your website
5. Look how often you are adding new content
6. Compare content you offer versus your competitors
7. Count the number of backlinks you have
8. Look up the age of your domain name and website.
9. Make sure you are listed on Google Maps.

Want to grow your local business? Start with online visibility!

The goal of your orthodontic practice SEO campaign is to boost rankings, traffic and conversions. SEO is much more than just adding a few keywords here and there to achieve a high ranking. Effective SEO requires continuous optimization. Working with a reputable orthodontic SEO firm is the key to getting the bookings you desire from new patients.

CHAPTER 8
HOW YOUR COMPETITORS INCREASE THEIR CONVERSION RATES

Is there another orthodontic practice in town that always seems to be one step ahead of you? It really makes you scratch your head and wonder what they are doing that you aren't. Is that orthodontist extra charismatic? Is his office more inviting? Does he offer better service? Or maybe his website is more professional. You notice that:

- Their website is amazing and loads super-fast.
- The pictures of his office look inviting.
- His ads seem to be everywhere online.
- Their website views much better on a smartphone than yours
- Their website ranks higher in Google than yours
- They have way more followers on Facebook than your practice

It could be that your competitor just has better conversion rates. Here we'll share the trends and insights you need to keep you on top and boost conversion.

Why Conversion Matters

Designing an ad that will draw in potential orthodontic patients is important. As an orthodontist, you don't need an extensive marketing background to do your job. However, some marketing knowledge can make the difference between a booming practice and just scraping by. When you track and analyze the results of your marketing campaigns you can figure out exactly what works and what doesn't work.

What Exactly Are Conversion Rates?

What exactly does have better conversion rates mean? Your conversion rate is the percentage of visitors to your website or landing page that convert to sales. Basically, that means that when a visitor goes to a website that it's more likely to convert that lead into a patient for your practice.

No two ads, social posts, or websites are alike. There are a number of tweaks you can make that result in increasing (or decreasing) the conversion rate. There's a lot more to putting together a successful ad than one that looks and sounds great. It's all about testing, tracking and tweaking till you get a good conversion rate.

Marketing Elements to Track for Effectiveness

After you launch your website, you want to track if it's really helping you attract new patients and increasing the demand for your services. There are specific landing pages that you send traffic to. You have signups for your mailing list. There are sequential email messages that you send once people sign up for your mailing list. You have calls to action at the bottom of every web page. There are different testimonials on your web pages. You have photographs. And there is copywriting on each of your web pages.

Wow! That's a lot more marketing elements then you probably thought about. It makes sense if you want to send leads to these marketing items you want to ensure that they get the best conversion. Your conversion rate describes how good your marketing is at getting people to do what you want them to do. You need to know how many people accept your offer compared to the number of people who visit your website.

Benefits of Boosting Your Conversion Rate

The number of benefits to boosting your conversion are massive! Boosting conversion rates can have a huge impact on your bottom line, so there are tons of benefits of conversion rate optimization. It can help your marketing dollars go farther. If you take the time to track and boost your conversion rate it will make your orthodontic practice more profitable.

Calculate Conversion Rate

In order to calculate your conversion rate, you just divide the number of conversions you get in a given time frame by the total number of people who visited your site or landing page and multiply it by 100%.

$$\textbf{\textit{Conversion rate = (conversions / total visitors) * 100\%}}$$

Website Elements to Boost Conversion

Conversion rate optimization involves testing multiple versions of different elements on your web site (like buttons, forms and calls to action/CTA) to determine which is the most effective in converting your visitors. Then, you can implement the best version and move on to testing another element.

There are a number of actions that you can track conversion rates on for your website. A good conversion rate should be around 3% to 5%. Some potential CTA's are:

- Call for information - List your phone number/general information.
- Schedule appointments - Share how to call or book an appointment online.
- Join mailing list - Have a form that visitors can fill out to join your mailing list.

- Downloading a free gift or report - This could be a free gift card for new patients.

- Sharing a page on social media – For instance, sharing a blog article on Facebook.

- Engaging with your site in some way (time on site, repeat visits, number of pages visited).

Offsite Elements to Test and Track

While some of the marketing elements you will want to enhance will be on your website, other elements that need to be improved may be off site items. For instance, your receptionist may be rude or not effective at booking appointments. There may be confusion about your appointment book that needs to be cleared up to make booking simpler. Maybe your wait times are running long. In short, make sure the patient experience is great from every angle.

The first step in tracking conversions is choosing what you want to track. For example, when you run ads with Google Ads, you may want to see whether clicks on your ad led a customer to take a certain action, such as booking an appointment, calling your office or signing up for a newsletter.

Web analytics is the measurement, collection, analysis and reporting of web data for purposes of understanding and optimizing web usage. Web analytics tools can meet your need for a comprehensive and filtered view to help you determine how users utilize digital channels such as the Web, mobile Internet and social media.

Below is a list of social media channels that offer analytics tools.

- Google Ads
- Google Analytics
- Facebook Ads (includes Instagram Ads)
- Twitter Ads
- Pinterest Promoted Pins

Google Analytics can be hooked up to your website to track conversions.

With good use of tracking numbers, codes, and other tools, you can reasonably measure the number of new patients generated by a specific campaign. Google Analytics helps you track keyword rank, pageviews and bounce rate while social media metrics help you track followers, social reach, engagement and conversions.

What Needs Testing

What should you test? Test everything! Sometimes the hardest part of A/B testing is determining what to test in the first place.

When you are testing elements of your marketing there's a lot of items that could be adjusted such as color, placement and images. You may need to increase the whitespace. Adding subheadings can help your text to be more easily scannable. Selective use of color can help readers move through your text. Your phone number may need to be in a bigger font.

Other items to try and adjust are adding your photo to the home page and a short welcome video.

Simplify the elements on your page. A confused mind says no. Try reducing distractions and options on your page so it's easier to read and take action.

Calls to action lead potential patients who visit your website to the pages you ultimately want them to view and complete a task on. Here are some examples:

- Schedule Appointment Now
- Schedule Online
- Request an Appointment
- Request a Virtual Consultation
- Call Our Emergency Hotline
- Read More
- See Testimonials
- Send My Free Report
- Email Us
- Map & Directions

Testing Color

Selecting color for your orthodontic website is important. Colors have qualities that can cause certain emotions in people. They influence an individual's decision-making and perceptions of your orthodontic practice. That is why choosing the right color for your orthodontic website is important to make a good first impression on potential patients. Here are a few to consider:

- Blue has always been a popular choice for orthodontic websites. Blue is the color of trust and intelligence. (Even Facebook uses it!) That trust and comfort conveys to patients that they will be in good hands.
- White is clean, honest, modern and transparent. This color exudes light and purity.

- Brown orthodontic websites give a feeling of home and comfort. For instance, if you are a specialist in sedation orthodontics, a brown decor may comfort your nervous patients.

- The color green communicates organic and holistic. If you are eco-friendly and conscious about the planet, this color will reveal that psychologically to your patients.

Use red sparingly. Most patients would faint at the thought or sight of blood at their orthodontic appointment. So, refrain from using that on your website or marketing materials.

Testing Methods.

One simple way to test is to use a focus group. They can do a usability test to work out the quirks. They will spot the typos, find the broken links, point out wording that doesn't make sense and alert you to questions that are not addressed.

Another way to test is with an A/B test. A/B testing (also sometimes referred to as split testing) is the practice of showing two versions of the same web page to different groups of visitors at the same time and comparing which version drives more conversions. You learn something about your visitors regardless of which variation wins.

For instance, I could do this with an ad testing two different headlines:

1. *Relaxing, Gentle, No Fear orthodontics*
2. *Relax and Be Comfortable with Sedation orthodontics.*

Show each ad to 100 people and see which one gets the most patients to book an appointment.

Conversion optimization is a crucial technique you need to survive in ultra-competitive markets

All marketing activities offline and online can have a tremendous impact on how your orthodontic marketing performs. Conversion optimization helps you to scrutinize what marketing activities you are conducting, what impact they are having and how to develop better experiences throughout the customer journey.

Some of your visitors end up buying from your competitors. If you don't have a strategy for winning in spite of competitors, you are doomed. It makes sense to have an expert review your website performance and offer recommendations. There are many ways to track your website's performance both online and offline, enabling you to measure its effectiveness.

It's not too late for you to jump ahead of your competition. As soon as they implement something, get ahead of the curve and use the opportunity to come out with the next big thing. Hopefully, this will inspire you to generate test ideas you can implement on your own website.

CHAPTER 9
THE RISKS OF DIY MARKETING

Marketing is an essential part of growing your orthodontic practice. After all, how hard could marketing be? At face value the do-it-yourself (DIY) route appears to offer a lot of savings but is it the right thing to do? Granted you may be marketing your orthodontic practice on your own to save money. But there are a lot of hidden costs to DIY marketing and it could be costing you a lot of business.

Let's look at the truth about marketing your orthodontic practice online on your own and some of the myths that come with it.

Myth #1

"I can just buy a how-to guide to get started. I'll just buy a book or take an online course to get up to speed. Anything you want to learn, there's a resource to learn that online."

The truth is your lack of knowledge and experience may cause you to do things incorrectly or inefficiently in a way that stifles your results. When you hire a professional, they are devoted to staying on top of changes in the industry. Their expertise allows them to achieve significantly better results than an amateur could.

SEO, email marketing, social media, pay per click and blogging are fast moving industries. Even the experts go to seminars, read constantly, and train to stay on top of their game. Plus, they have real world experience working with other clients on all aspects of marketing. Whatever your challenge or question, they will know how to handle it.

Myth #2

"I am saving money by doing it myself. It's costly to hire a marketing agency."

To create a brilliant campaign, you need to be a copywriter, graphic designer, social media expert, strategist, software guru and more. Marketing teams provide these skills and expertise under one umbrella. The truth is that when you skimp on marketing, you may get lackluster results. DIY marketing isn't as cost-effective as you may imagine.

A marketing team knows best practices and how to maximize your budget. Now imagine the money you could potentially spend on a pay per click campaign that doesn't convert well. If a professional designed and tested the same ad they could generate a lot of more leads on the same advertising budget.

Myth #3

"I know what content my customers want. I talk to my patients every day."

Advertising and content marketing have proven to be insanely effective and can be integral to building the trust that inevitably leads to conversions. Content marketing isn't something you want to jump

into blindly. You want to ensure cohesiveness, to express brand identity, and to review patterns for popular content. You need to have a strategic marketing plan that aligns your content with your sales promotions. Then you need to compose posts and marketing messages in a way that converts leads.

Myth #4

"I know a bit about Local SEO and it's not that hard to implement."

Local search engine optimization (SEO) is crucial to enable your website to rank well in the search engines like Google, Yahoo and Bing. With the constant changes in the way Google indexes web pages, it can be challenging to stay on the first page of results. Doing it yourself could result in targeting the wrong keywords. In fact, there may be keywords that generate a lot more traffic and get better results. There's a lot to know about local SEO. If you do it wrong, you could actually get your website blacklisted. It's imperative that your search engine optimization is done both correctly and cost-effectively.

Myth #5

"Social media is easy. Just write and post. No big deal."

You could set up a Facebook Page, an Instagram and a Twitter account, start posting and hope for the best, or you could actually strategize and achieve success on social media. While DIY social media marketing can be a cost-effective approach in the beginning, recovering from mistakes can be extremely costly in the long run. Everything done in social media; from the post times, to location settings, to engagement strategies, all require research, strategy and again, intention.

Myth #6

"I can handle my own email marketing. Just write, click, send. No big deal."

If you're DIYing it with email right now, you may be sitting on some untapped potential revenue. The failure most DIY marketers make with email marketing is that they write a sales pitch that is focused on them. In order for your emails to be opened, actually read, and shared they need to be written with what's in it for the reader. It has to be personal and connective. It has to be focused on how you can help them.

Myth #7

"I have time to manage my own marketing campaigns. Or I can have one of my staff members do it."

When you're running an orthodontic practice, time is a precious commodity, and marketing your brand can take up plenty of your time. Every hour you spend on marketing is time that you are not spending on income generating activities like taking care of patients. Having a staff member handle, it means that they are not taking care of essential orthodontic business tasks. You steal away a few hours each week to concentrate on DIY marketing instead of focusing on your core responsibilities. This divided attention can have a negative impact on other areas of your orthodontic practice. Outsourcing to a marketing professional frees you to focus on what you do best: work with patients.

Myth #8

"I can write my own blog posts. After all, I am an expert in orthodontics."

Blogging is one of the best ways to drive inbound traffic and convert visitors into leads. If you're making the common mistakes that many newbie bloggers make, your traffic will suffer. Your orthodontist blog has to be high quality and relevant enough to bring in traffic and capture leads.

Although you are an orthodontic expert, you might not be writing about the topics your audience cares about most. Or you may be writing above their heads. You probably aren't SEO optimizing your blog posts properly. Finally, you may not be including calls to action in your blog posts.

Myth #9

"I can create my own website with a predesigned orthodontic website template."

To conserve funds, some orthodontic practices will want to design their first website on their own. Unfortunately, DIY business website design is a terrible idea in most cases. By hiring a professional web designer or agency, you ensure that your orthodontic practice website serves the needs of your business. Your website must attract visitors, engage them and convert them into patients right from the start. Doing this on your own will take a lot of trial and error and most likely, you will not succeed on your own.

The Big Picture

So, let's review some of the DIY Fails you will experience by handling your own marketing

Underwhelming results - You don't have time to monitor social media. You don't know how to monitor search engine rankings. You are too busy to spend proper time marketing.

Lack of understanding of the target audience - You have an idea of what kind of clients you want, but the clients you are attracting are very different from that idea.

Not having up to date knowledge and experience in online marketing - Admit your expertise is orthodontics, not online marketing.

Lost income because you focused on marketing and not your core business - When you can bill several hundred dollars per hour for orthodontic work, it really is costly for you to spend your own time on marketing.

Unfocused marketing campaigns - Admittedly, you post whatever great idea of the moment you have and don't have a cohesive marketing plan that guides your marketing efforts.

Lower conversion rates for advertising campaigns - You do the best you can with what you know. But there are tips, tricks and best practices you don't know that affect your marketing results.

Lost traffic because of use of wrong keywords - You optimize for phrases that seem important but don't have research tools to strategically select what you optimize for.

Poor quality content - Okay. You are not a writer. But I bet if a marketer interviewed you on specific topics, they could get knowledge to write a targeted article in language that your prospects understand.

Not having enough time to devote to marketing activities - You don't want to spend lunch hours or family time doing social posts. Outsource it and protect your personal time as well as avoid making costly mistakes due to not having an up to date knowledge of marketing. Now let's look at the benefits of **outsourcing** your marketing.

An outside point of view - It can be eye opening to have an outside agency take a look at your marketing plans to find new and innovative ideas you haven't thought of.

Access to the latest technology - They have tools and technology that help them do tasks efficiently and more precisely.

Cutting edge marketing expertise - Your marketing team actively researches, creates and implements marketing strategies that work. Online marketing experts spend most of their time learning new skills and improving on existing techniques and strategies.

Consistency - Interacting with consumers through a consistent brand voice and aesthetic is a major step towards letting consumers get to know you as an organization.

Greater bandwidth to scale up marketing efforts - You have access to an entire team of people to employ your campaign.

Improve focus on strategy and execution - They are on top of the most up-to-date tactics and trends to find your best customers and develop a truly effective strategy.

Ongoing optimization of campaigns - Your marketing team constantly reviews statistics of your marketing campaign and adjusts to ensure best results. They're genuinely interested in, and committed to, continually optimizing your strategy for best results.

Deliver greater results and ROI - Your marketing agency will spend time making sure you get the results you paid for.

Lower overhead versus having a full-time marketer on staff - It's expensive to have an in-house marketing team.

How to Find and Hire the Right Marketing Agency for You

There are a number of critical things to consider before making the leap and hiring a firm that will save you money, time and headaches.

Review the Agency's Case Studies. Don't just go by the testimonials on their agency website. Any agency worth their salt should be able and willing to share a case study with you. Look for an agency with experience in orthodontic or orthodontic marketing, but also one who can prove (and guarantee?) they can get you results.

Take advantage of a free consultation. You want someone you can talk with who genuinely listens and can respond to your concerns. Be sure to ask in advance what they provide. What does it cost? How much is included in your base fee?

Try them on a test project before you sign a longer contract. You want to know what the experience of working with them is like and if they generate the results they promise.

We've already debunked the idea that DIY marketing saves money. Do you really want to spend more of your valuable time trying to educate yourself on DIY marketing when qualified experts are standing by? The planning, training, and educational benefits of working with a marketing expert can make a dramatic difference in your marketing results. It's time to see what's possible when you let the experts handle your marketing. Just sit back, let them do the work, and watch the patients come in.

CHAPTER 10

THE ULTIMATE

ONLINE MARKETING CHECKLIST

- Do you have a website?

- Is it properly optimized for search?
  - Do you have your main keyword in the title tag on each of the pages of your website?
  - Do you have pages for each of your core services?
  - Do you have pages for the solutions that you service in your business?
  - Do you have unique content on each of the pages of your website?
  - Are you helping Google understand your true service area?

- Does your website rank on page one for your most important keywords like "your city + business", "your city + service", "your city + pain point"?

- Is your website optimized for conversion (visitors to callers)?
  - Do you have the phone number in the top right corner on every page?
  - Are you using authentic images / video? Photo of the team, photo of your office, photo of your team, etc?
  - Do you have a compelling call to action after ever block of text?

- Is your website mobile-friendly?

- Are you consistently creating new content, blogging to create new inbound organic links back to your website?

- Have you optimized correctly for the Google Map Listings?

- Are you consistently creating new content, blogging to create new inbound organic links back to your website?
  - Are you on all the major online directory listings with the same company name, address & phone number?
  - How many online reviews do you have?
  - Do you have a proactive strategy for getting new online reviews every day?

o **Are you active on social media?**

o **Are you leveraging email marketing for current or future clients?**
   - o Do you have a database with your customer email addresses?
   - o Are you sending out a monthly email newsletter?
   - o Are you leveraging email to get online reviews & to draw customers into your social media profiles?

o **Are you taking advantage of paid online marketing opportunities?**
   - o Do you have a Google Ads Campaign? Are you strategically targeting with specific ad groups, text ads & landing pages?

o **Do you have the proper tracking in place to gauge your ROI?**
   - o Google Analytics
   - o Keyword Ranking Tracking
   - o Call Tracking
   - o CRM with tracked lead sources
   - o Google Search Console

NEXT STEP FOR YOUR PRACTICE
DO THIS RIGHT NOW!

Now that you know what to do, and how to do it… it's time for you to take action.

In writing this book I set out to provide real value to you and provide strategies and ideas that you could actually use in your own marketing efforts and apply them to your practice, and I think I managed to do that, but this book is of no value to you if you don't apply any of it.

My hope is that you will go and apply, even some of this information and see results for yourself.

If you aren't sure you want to do this yourself, and you want to reach out to get further customized help, the offer is there.

I'll leave my links below for your convenience. But in any event, if you don't end up working with us, still go ahead and apply what you've learned from this book.

We Guarantee Results, Or You Don't Pay!!

It's just that simple.

Schedule a call with me at the link below, and if you end up working with us, mentioning this book will get you $100 towards our services.

https://orthoadvertising.com/book-a-call

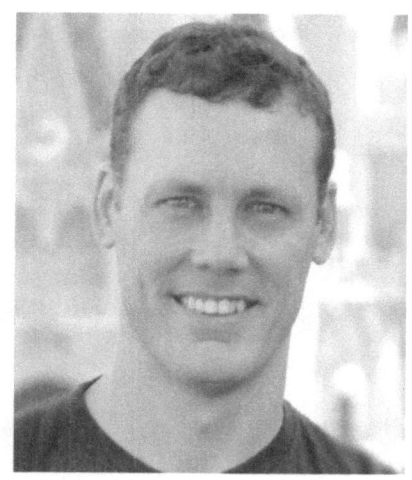

Adam Roseland is the founder of **Ortho Advertising** (https://orthoadvertising.com), an award winning Philadelphia based Digital Marketing Agency providing expert SEO, Google Ads, Facebook & Instagram Ads Management & Retargeting.

Adam has been working in the advertising industry for the past 20 years, primarily in the digital space, helping local practices get more patients and creating one of the industry's leading search marketing companies.

Bonus for SEO – Best Places To Build Backlinks:

Create Backlinks to your practice website with any of the following:

VIDEO BACKLINKS

http://www.youtube.com
http://www.vimeo.com
http://www.dailymotion.com
http://www.twitch.tv
http://www.flickr.com
http://www.ustream.tv
https://tune.pk

Add your link on "about", "info" or "channel" page

PHOTOGRAPHY BACKLINKS

http://www.flickr.com
http://www.istockphoto.com
http://www.shutterstock.com
http://www.dreamstime.com
https://unsplash.com

Sells pictures on all the stock photography site. Include a link back to your main site on your profile page.

TALK SHOW / DJ BACKLINKS

http://itunes.apple.com
http://soundcloud.com
http://www.mixcloud.com

Add links to your podcast and / or profile

MUSIC BACKLINKS
http://www.purevolume.com
http://www.soundclick.com

Create blog post commenting with backlink and / or add account backlink

BE TALKATIVE BACKLINKS
http://disqus.com
http://www.ted.com
http://reddit.com

Add profile or comment backlinks

SOCIAL BACKLINKS
http://pinterest.com
http://twitter.com
http://www.reddit.com
http://stumbleupon.com
https://www.vk.com
http://www.tumblr.com
http://www.myspace.com

Gain backlinks from main profile page, individual posts and leaving "likes" / "upvotes"

COMMUNITY BACKLINKS
http://groups.yahoo.com
http://wikia.com

Set profile link and / or include links on sub-pages

GRAPHIC BACKLINKS
http://visual.ly/view
http://storify.com
https://www.behance.net/
https://about.me

Add profile, reference & sources backlinks

ILLUSTRATION BACKLINKS

http://submitinfographics.com/
http://coolinfographics.com/contact/
http://infographicjournal.com/submit-infographics/
http://infographicsarchive.com/submit-infographics/
http://infographicplaza.com/submit-infographics/
http://topinfographic.com/index.php/submit-infographics/
http://www.infographicsshowcase.com/submit/
http://theinfographics.blogspot.co.uk/p/submit-infographic_22.html
http://www.best-infographics.com/product/first-day-service/
http://www.infographicpost.com/submit-an-infographic

Share your infographics that cover important topics in your niche

FAN CLUB BACKLINKS

https://groups.diigo.com/index
https://www.facebook.com

Create a fan page and include a public link in the info

CONTENT CURATION BACKLINKS

http://www.scoop.it/
https://about.flipboard.com/tools/

Curating relevant content together. Include your own content for links back

ACADEMIC PAPERS BACKLINKS

http://academia.edu
http://www.springer.com/gp/#c35020
http://www.elsevier.com/journal-authors/home#submit-paper

Own profile and research paper article links

CONTRIBUTE TO MAN KIND BACKLINKS

http://wikipedia.com
http://thefullwiki.org
http://www.wikihow.com

Fix entries & add references with your papers

DISTRIBUTE SOFTWARE BACKLINKS

http://download.com
http://portableapps.com
http://freewarefiles.com
http://tucows.com
http://www.softpedia.com
http://filehippo.com
http://www.soft32.com
http://www.snapfiles.com
http://www.brothersoft.com

Submit your application & add a profile backlink

SCHOLARSHIP BACKLINKS

https://www.southalabama.edu/departments/financialaffairs/scholarships/externalscholarshipsa-z.html
http://www.oll.usouthal.edu/departments/financialaffairs/scholarships/externalscholarshipsa-z.html
http://www.tarleton.edu/scholarships/outsideresources.html
http://www.uh.edu/financial/undergraduate/types-aid/scholarships
http://www.marquette.edu/mucentral/financialaid/resources_pvt_scholar_misc.shtml
https://www.ndscs.edu/paying-for-college/scholarships/available-external-scholarships
http://www.daemen.edu/admissions/affordability/financial-aid/external-scholarships
http://louisville.edu/financialaid/scholarships/outside-scholarships.html
https://ldsbc.edu/scholarship-information/outside-scholarships.html
http://www.spcollege.edu/private-donor-scholarships
http://www.callutheran.edu/financial-aid/scholarships-grants/outside-scholarships.html
http://www.hawkeyecollege.edu/financial-aid/types-of-aid/grants-and-scholarships/scholarships.aspx
http://www.westliberty.edu/financial-aid/outside-scholarships
https://www.mtmc.edu/tuition-and-aid/financing-your-education/scholarships-andawards/outside-scholarships/outside-resources

Set up a scholarship page on your site and inform the following universities so they can add it on their site.

REQUEST TECHNICAL HELP BACKLINKS

http://wordpress.org/support/topic
http://help.com
http://www.sitepoint.com/forums/
https://groups.google.com/forum/#!forum/feedburner
https://bugzilla.mozilla.org/
https://forum.joomla.org/
Request help about "problems" on your site - add link to your site

HELP A REPORTER BACKLINKS

http://haro.com
http://www.responsesource.com
http://www.prnewswire.com/profnet/
http://www.sourcebottle.com
http://mediakitty.com

Help journalists with their stories and get referenced in return

BECOME AN AUTHOR BACKLINKS

https://theconversation.com/become-an-author
https://www.forbes.com/fdc/contact.html
http://elitedaily.com/contribute/
https://www.entrepreneur.com/page/236106
https://tnw.typeform.com/to/Wxbs5j
http://www.inquisitr.com/write-for-inquisitr/
http://technical.ly/contributor-form/
http://www.cultbox.co.uk/write-for-us
http://www.businesszone.co.uk/guidelines-for-features-on-businesszonecouk
http://www.business2community.com/become-a-contributor
http://www.shoemoney.com/shoemoney-author-application/
http://www.lifehack.org/contribute
http://www.business2community.com/become-a-contributor
http://www.bizcommunity.com/SubmitNews.aspx?l=196&c=11
http://www.iamwire.com/submit-guest-post
https://www.techwyse.com/write-for-us/
https://smallbiztrends.com/contribute-articles
http://www.socialmediaexaminer.com/writers/

Become an author on respected sites. Contribute by writing articles and leaving backlinks within content for maximum juice

ACQUIRING AUTHORS BACKLINKS

http://fiverr.com
http://upwork.com
http://peopleperhour.com
http://konker.io
http://mentionade.com
Use the following services to find authors who will write for you and add a link on established websites / blogs

OUTREACH EXPERTS BACKLINKS

http://posirank.com/eric/
http://thehoth.com
http://fatjoe.co/blogger-outreach/

Use services to find guest bloggers & writers

DONATIONS BACKLINKS

http://xchat.org/donate/
http://www.apache.org/foundation/thanks.html
https://www.phpmyadmin.net/sponsors/
https://creativecommons.org/supporters/
http://www.awstats.org/awstats_supporters.php
http://www.opensourcecms.com/support/halloffame.php
http://www.opencms-days.org/sponsors/our-sponsors/
http://events.linuxfoundation.org/events/openiot-summit/sponsors/our-sponsors

Get rewarded with a link for your sizeable donation

HOST AN EVENT BACKLINKS

https://www.eventbrite.com/
http://meetup.com/
https://www.metooo.io

Create an event along with crafted related content around your link

CERTIFICATIONS & REVIEWS BACKLINKS

http://bbb.org
http://yelp.com
http://www.google.com/business/
https://smallbusiness.yahoo.com/local-listings
http://www.dmca.com

PUBLISH PRESENTATIONS BACKLINKS

http://scribd.com
http://docs.google.com
http://slideshare.net
http://www.authorstream.com
http://www.issuu.com
https://speakerdeck.com

Add links within your presentation & profile

COMPANY OVERVIEW BACKLINKS

http://trello.com

Create a public board for your company / niche. Add link back to your website with contextual information around it / leave a link in your profile

QUESTION & ANSWER BACKLINKS

http://askville.amazon.com
http://answers.yahoo.com
http://www.quora.com
http://www.blurtit.com/
https://www.fluther.com

Answer questions and include a link in it / add link to your profile

PRESS RELEASE BACKLINKS

http://prweb.com
http://prnewswire.com

Different press releases get onto different sites and provide different type of backlinks

PUBLISHING GUIDES BACKLINKS
http://guides.co/

Create a new guide and include reference links inside

START A PROJECT BACKLINKS
https://github.com/
Create a programming project.

The links inside your readme file are readable links

PROVIDE TECHNICAL HELP BACKLINKS
https://answers.microsoft.com/en-us

Answer questions from the community & add links to your site

200 Social Profiles Every Business Should Create:

https://social.msdn.microsoft.com/
https://forums.adobe.com/people/
https://www.behance.net/
https://www.imdb.com/user/ur100519086
https://revolistsg.blogspot.com/
https://www.amazon.com/gp/profile/
https://www.skillshare.com/
https://myspace.com/
http://digg.com/
https://sites.google.com/
https://www.codementor.io/
https://disqus.com/
https://able2know.org/
https://profiles.wordpress.org/
https://justpaste.it/
https://www.curbed.com/
https://www.couchsurfing.com/
https://starlocalmedia.com/
https://www.kdpcommunity.com/
https://wordpress.com/
https://www.sidefx.com/
https://www.designspiration.net/
https://www.eater.com/
https://www.pozible.com/
https://en.gravatar.com/
https://www.beezmap.com/
https://gust.com/
https://www.theverge.com/
https://photoshopcreative.co.uk/
https://kinja.com/
http://www.koinup.com/
https://knowyourmeme.com/
https://www.sbnation.com/
https://www.viki.com/

http://proboards.com/
http://www.measuredup.com/
https://www.redbubble.com/
https://growthhackers.com/
https://www.patreon.com/
http://wallinside.com/
https://www.bloglovin.com/
https://www.hackerrank.com/
https://www.racked.com/
https://www.empowher.com/
http://www.articles.gappoo.com/
http://www.alternion.com/
https://weheartit.com/
https://www.concertwindow.com/
https://www.creativelive.com/
http://bravesites.com/
https://www.cnet.com/
https://ello.co/
https://www.artfire.com/
https://www.funnyordie.com/
https://wixsite.com/
https://www.easel.ly/
https://giphy.com/
https://www.kickstarter.com/
https://www.slideserve.com/
https://posteezy.com/
https://www.free-ebooks.net/
https://www.deviantart.com/
https://www.twitch.tv/
https://www.4shared.com/
http://wikidot.com
http://ttlink.com/
https://www.crunchyroll.com/
https://www.recode.net/
https://globegazette.com/
http://freeforums.net/

https://globegazette.com/
https://soundcloud.com/
https://mix.com/
https://techspy.com/
http://boards.net/
https://www.gapyear.com/
https://coub.com/
https://nus.academia.edu/
http://www.plerb.com/
https://fastlisting.org/
https://guides.co/
https://visual.ly/
https://steepster.com/
https://snipplr.com/
http://www.articles.seoforums.me.uk/
https://sourceforge.net/
http://www.wittygraphy.com/
https://myanimelist.net/
https://sportspyder.com/
https://write.as/
https://cookpad.com/
https://itsmyurls.com/
https://www.blackplanet.com/
http://archive.is/
http://brandyourself.com/
https://steamcommunity.com/
https://www.colourlovers.com/
https://www.goodreads.com/
https://www.crowdfunder.co.uk/
https://jimdofree.com/
https://columbustelegram.com/
https://letterboxd.com/
https://www.ted.com/
http://profile.hatena.ne.jp/
http://www.articles.howto-tips.com/
http://www.mentionade.com/

https://www.plurk.com/

https://ask.fm/

https://my.desktopnexus.com/

https://ucraft.net

https://www.intensedebate.com/

https://www.slideshare.net/

http://www.seobook.com/

https://id.arduino.cc/

http://strikingly.com/

https://onmogul.com/

https://www.udemy.com/

https://stocktwits.com/

http://www.brijj.com/

https://cheezburger.com/

http://www.ihubbub.com/

https://devpost.com/

https://n4g.com/

http://dayviews.com/

https://paper.li/

https://www.gaiaonline.com/

https://creativemarket.com/

https://tinychat.com/

https://getpocket.com/

http://simplesite.com/

https://www.victoriaadvocate.com/

https://www.diigo.com/

https://tracky.com/

http://pin.anime.com/

https://sitey.me/

https://poptype.co/

https://www.crokes.com/

https://public.bookmax.net/

https://clarity.fm/

https://medium.com/

https://speakerdeck.com/

https://www.mixcloud.com/

https://picturepush.com/
https://slashdot.org/
http://www.articles.mybikaner.com/
https://www.smore.com/
https://500px.com/
https://getsatisfaction.com/
https://answers.informer.com/
http://moonfruit.com/
https://www.vox.com/
https://www.buzzfeed.com/
https://www.play.fm/
http://www.fotobabble.com/
https://yolasite.com/
http://www.datpiff.com/
http://qooh.me/
https://www.spreaker.com/
https://www.mindmeister.com/
http://postbits.net/
http://dojo.press/
https://www.edocr.com/
https://slides.com/
https://www.gamespot.com/
https://telegra.ph/
https://hubski.com/
http://www.authorstream.com/
http://www.magcloud.com/
https://www.hometalk.com/
https://carbonmade.com/
https://butterflycoins.org/
http://whazzup-u.com/
https://www.zomato.com/
http://www.blurb.com/
http://my-free.website/
https://wanelo.co/
https://www.minds.com/
https://www.wattpad.com/

https://www.codecademy.com/
http://jigsy.com/
https://www.wishlistr.com/
https://www.adsoftheworld.com/
https://www.instructables.com/
https://www.f6s.com/
http://www.articles.kraftloft.com/
http://www.fixya.com/
https://imgur.com/
https://dzone.com/
http://www.blogtalkradio.com/
https://livejournal.com/
https://www.kiva.org/
https://angel.co/
https://hubpages.com/
https://www.ifixit.com/
http://pen.io/
https://www.faceparty.com/
https://www.instapaper.com/
http://www.folkd.com/
https://remote.com/
https://weebly.com/
https://gurudb.com/